FROM MANAGING TO CONQUERING CYSTITIS

Expert Guide To Understanding Causes, Recognizing Symptoms, And Embracing Effective Treatment For A Path To Healthy Living

DR. DASHIELL DANIEL

Conquering Cystitis" is a landmark work in the field of urological health that offers a thorough examination of cystitis, a common and frequently incapacitating urinary tract condition. The book carefully looks at the various facets of cystitis, from its basic definitions and classifications to a thorough investigation of its causes and risk factors. The importance of this volume rests in its capacity to function as a vital educational tool for both medical professionals and patients suffering from cystitis, promoting a better comprehension of the condition's intricacies.

In the first few chapters, signs and symptoms are identified in detail, providing readers with the knowledge they need to identify the onset of cystitis. This diagnostic basis is then supplemented with a thorough analysis of various treatment options, ranging from traditional pharmaceutical interventions to holistic and alternative remedies. The book also covers lifestyle modifications, including dietary advice and hygiene practices, providing useful strategies for management and prevention.

One of "Conquering Cystitis"'s unique selling points is its diversity; it covers the ways in which cystitis manifests differently in women, men, and pediatric patients. This specialized approach enables a more nuanced comprehension of the ways in which the condition affects different groups of people, which in turn leads to more individualized and successful treatment plans.

In addition, the examination of coping strategies for chronic cystitis illuminates the psychological and emotional costs associated with the illness.

The book provides integration techniques and supportive strategies that enable a comprehensive management strategy for cystitis that goes beyond treating symptoms.

One of the book's most noteworthy aspects is its dedication to staying up to date with the most recent research and developments in the treatment of cystitis.

The final chapters offer an overview of the state of medical research, new treatments, and potential future paths in the field. As a result, "Conquering Cystitis" is not only a valuable reference book but also a living archive of knowledge that is constantly being updated, encouraging ongoing discussion in the quest for improved cystitis care.

Overview

Mostly brought on by bacterial infections, cystitis is a common inflammatory condition that affects the bladder. Despite being common, cystitis can cause a great deal of discomfort and distress for those who experience its symptoms. To effectively treat and overcome cystitis, it is important to have a thorough understanding of all of its aspects. This discussion will cover the definition and general overview of cystitis, as well as the various types of the condition and the complex web of causes and risk factors associated with this urinary tract ailment.

Comprehending Cystitis

A deeper understanding of cystitis entails understanding its underlying mechanisms, including the invasion of bacteria into the bladder, which is a primary causative factor. Additionally, understanding the role of the immune system in responding to the infection is crucial for developing effective therapeutic interventions. Above all, cystitis is primarily defined by inflammation of the bladder, a hollow muscular organ that is essential for storing and expelling urine from the body. When this organ becomes inflamed, it frequently presents as symptoms like frequent and painful urination, a persistent urge to urinate, and discomfort in the pelvic area.

Definition And Synopsis

An overview of cystitis includes taking into account its prevalence in different demographics, with women being more susceptible due to anatomical factors, and investigating the impact it can have on an individual's quality of life.

Cystitis is commonly defined as the inflammation of the bladder wall, usually resulting from a bacterial infection.

The inflammatory response triggered by the presence of bacteria leads to a range of symptoms, from mild discomfort to severe pain. The condition is often classified into two main types: infectious cystitis, which is primarily caused by bacterial invasion, and non-infectious cystitis, which may result from factors like irritants, radiation, or underlying medical conditions.

Cystitis Types

There are various forms of cystitis, each with unique traits and underlying causes. The most common type is infectious cystitis, which is often brought on by the bacteria Escherichia coli, which normally lives in the gastrointestinal tract but can enter the urethra and ascend into the bladder. Non-infectious cystitis, on the other hand, includes a range of conditions like chemical cystitis, radiation cystitis, and interstitial cystitis, all of which are brought on by different factors. Knowing the differences between these types is important for developing effective treatment plans. For example, interstitial cystitis involves persistent inflammation of the bladder wall without a clear infectious cause, making diagnosis difficult and necessitating specific management techniques.

Reasons And Danger Elements

The causes and risk factors associated with cystitis are multifaceted, encompassing a range of elements that contribute to the development of this inflammatory condition. Bacterial infections, particularly by Escherichia coli, are a primary cause of infectious cystitis. Understanding the mechanisms by which bacteria gain access to the bladder and evade the body's defense mechanisms is essential for preventive measures. Non-infectious cystitis, on the other hand, can be triggered by irritants such as certain medications, radiation therapy, or underlying medical conditions like bladder dysfunction. Moreover, gender differences play a significant role in the prevalence of cystitis, with women being more susceptible due to the proximity of the urethra to the anus. Other risk factors include age, sexual activity, urinary tract abnormalities, and the use of certain contraceptives. A comprehensive understanding of these causes and risk factors is imperative for effective prevention strategies and targeted treatment approaches.

the fight against cystitis necessitates a comprehensive grasp of all its facets, from the definition and general overview of the illness to the detailed investigation of its types and the complex causes and risk factors that contribute to its development. By thoroughly addressing each of these facets, medical professionals can develop focused interventions that not only reduce symptoms but also aid in the prevention and long-term management of cystitis.

CHAPTER ONE
IDENTIFYING THE SYMPTOMS AND SIGNS

Cystitis, also referred to as a urinary tract infection (UTI), is a common inflammatory bladder condition that affects millions of people worldwide. It is important to recognize the signs and symptoms of cystitis in order to effectively manage the condition and initiate early intervention. Symptoms of bladder inflammation typically include burning when urinating frequently, cloudy or strong-smelling urine, and occasionally, blood in the urine, which indicates the potential severity of the infection. Another common symptom of cystitis is lower abdominal discomfort or pain.

Common Cystitis Symptoms

Cystitis is a urinary tract infection that can cause a variety of symptoms, so it's important to understand the common ones that are associated with it. Those who develop cystitis typically experience increased frequency of urination along with a heightened urgency to empty the bladder. This frequent urge is often accompanied by dysuria, which is a painful or burning sensation during urination that can have a significant impact on an individual's quality of life. Additionally, changes in urine color and odor are common symptoms because cystitis can cause blood or pus to appear in the urine, giving it a cloudy appearance and a distinct smell. Recognizing these symptoms can help both individuals and healthcare providers diagnose and treat cystitis in a timely manner.

When To Get Medical Help

It is critical to know when to seek medical attention for cystitis in order to prevent complications and ensure that the infection resolves quickly. When it comes to cystitis, there are a few signs that call for prompt medical attention: blood in the urine, severe pelvic pain, fever, chills, and other systemic symptoms that may indicate a more serious infection or potential complications and call for immediate medical attention. Pregnant women, people with pre-existing health conditions, and people who have a history of recurrent UTIs should also be cautious about seeking prompt medical evaluation.

Identifying Cystitis

Accurate diagnosis of cystitis is crucial for implementing appropriate treatment strategies and preventing the progression of the infection. Healthcare professionals employ a combination of clinical evaluation, medical history assessment, and diagnostic tests to confirm the presence of cystitis. During the clinical assessment, healthcare providers inquire about the nature and duration of symptoms, any previous history of UTIs, and potential risk factors. Urinalysis is a fundamental diagnostic tool, allowing for the examination of urine for signs of infection, such as the presence of bacteria, white blood cells, and red blood cells. In some cases, urine cultures may be conducted to identify the specific causative bacteria and guide antibiotic therapy. Imaging studies, such as ultrasound or cystoscopy, may be recommended in certain situations to assess the extent of bladder involvement or rule out other underlying conditions. A comprehensive and accurate diagnosis ensures targeted and effective management, reducing the risk of recurrence and complications associated with cystitis.

CHAPTER TWO
ANALYZING POSSIBLE TREATMENTS

Cystitis, also referred to as a urinary tract infection (UTI), is a common and uncomfortable condition that affects a significant portion of the population, particularly women. When treating cystitis, it is important to investigate various treatment options to provide effective and targeted relief.

One primary avenue involves the use of antibiotics and medications. Antibiotics, such as trimethoprim-sulfamethoxazole, nitrofurantoin, and ciprofloxacin, are frequently prescribed to combat bacterial infections that cause cystitis.

These medications function by identifying and eradicating the causative bacteria, which helps to relieve symptoms and promote recovery. However, the emergence of antibiotic resistance emphasizes the need for caution when using antibiotics and to consider alternative treatment options.

At-Home Treatments For Pain

Home remedies are an important part of the treatment plan in addition to conventional medical interventions. Drinking more water helps flush out bacteria from the urinary system and promote healing. Cranberry juice, well known for its UTI-prevention properties, may help relieve symptoms by preventing bacteria from adhering to the urinary tract lining.

Maintaining good hygiene, including regular voiding and proper genital care, can prevent the worsening of cystitis. Including probiotics in the diet helps maintain a healthy balance of gut bacteria, which may lower the risk of recurrent infections. Nevertheless, one should be cautious and seek medical advice before relying solely on home remedies for cystitis.

Techniques For Pain Management

Effective pain management strategies are necessary because cystitis frequently causes discomfort and pain, making it difficult for affected individuals to lead fulfilling lives. Nonsteroidal anti-inflammatory drugs (NSAIDs), like ibuprofen, can be used to reduce pain and inflammation associated with cystitis. These medications work by inhibiting prostaglandin synthesis, which in turn reduces the inflammatory response.

However, individuals with contraindications or pre-existing conditions should use caution when using NSAIDs because they may have negative effects on renal function and gastrointestinal health. Additionally, applying heat, using hot water bottles or warm baths, can help provide localized relief by relieving the affected area and encouraging muscle relaxation. Behavioral interventions, such as

the complex nature of cystitis necessitates a multimodal approach to treatment. While antibiotics and medications are still essential for eliminating bacterial infections, the growing concern about antibiotic resistance highlights the need for alternative approaches. Home remedies are a useful supplement to traditional treatments, focusing on prevention and overall health.

Pain management strategies, including both pharmaceutical and non-pharmacological interventions, are critical for improving the comfort and quality of life for those with cystitis.

By combining these various treatment options, medical professionals can customize their care to each patient's specific requirements, ensuring efficient relief and a reduced chance of recurrence.

CHAPTER THREE
MODIFICATIONS TO LIFESTYLE FOR PREVENTION

The prevention and management of cystitis, a common urinary tract infection (UTI), entails a multimodal approach that includes lifestyle modifications to lower the risk of recurrence. Lifestyle modifications are essential to preserving urinary tract health and preventing the onset of cystitis. People who are predisposed to UTIs frequently experience relief from episodes and a reduction in the frequency of episodes through lifestyle modifications. These modifications include dietary changes, hygiene practices, and urinary habits. Together, these modifications form part of a comprehensive strategy for the prevention of cystitis, which emphasizes a proactive and holistic approach to urinary health.

The Dietary Guidelines

In order to prevent and manage cystitis, one must make certain dietary choices. Some foods and beverages can either exacerbate symptoms or act as protective agents against bacterial infections. Eating a well-balanced diet with plenty of fruits, vegetables, and whole grains provides essential nutrients that support the immune system.

Drinking more water is a key recommendation because it helps flush out bacteria from the urinary tract and promotes hydration. On the other hand, avoiding certain irritants, like caffeine and acidic foods, can be helpful because they may worsen symptoms or cause cystitis to recur.

Hygienic Habits

The prevention of cystitis and its recurrence depends on maintaining good hygiene practices. The urethra's close proximity to the anus creates an environment in which bacteria can easily enter the urinary tract and cause infections.

Regular and thorough cleansing of the genital area, especially before and after sexual activity, is critical in minimizing the risk of bacterial entry. Avoiding harsh or irritating soaps, bubble baths, and feminine hygiene products that may upset the natural balance of the genital microbiota is advised. Furthermore, maintaining good hand hygiene, including proper handwashing techniques, is essential in preventing the spread of bacteria from hands to the urinary tract.

These hygiene practices constitute a cornerstone in the preventive measures against

Urinary Behaviors

A crucial part of preventing cystitis is developing healthy urinary habits. People can reduce their risk of urinary tract infections (UTIs) by implementing strategies that encourage regular and complete bladder emptying. These include not holding off on urinating when they have the urge and making sure they give their bladder enough time to empty completely.

Women, in particular, should use proper wiping techniques after using the toilet to prevent the transfer of bacteria from the anus to the urethra. Additionally, urinating before and after sexual activity can help flush out bacteria that may have entered the urethra during sexual activity. Adequate hydration promotes urinary health by diluting urine and making it easier to eliminate bacteria.

Finally, a holistic strategy for cystitis prevention emphasizes the significance of maintaining a balanced and health-conscious approach to one's daily habits. The prevention of cystitis entails a comprehensive approach that includes lifestyle modifications, including dietary modifications, hygiene practices, and urinary habits.

By understanding the interplay between these factors, individuals can proactively manage their urinary health and reduce the frequency of cystitis episodes.

CHAPTER FOUR
INTEGRATIVE METHODS FOR TREATING CYSTITIS

Cystitis is an inflammatory bladder condition that frequently manifests as symptoms like urgency, frequency, and discomfort. Holistic approaches to treating cystitis are multifaceted and go beyond traditional medical interventions. One aspect of holistic care that stands out is the incorporation of herbal remedies. Herbal remedies have been used for centuries in many cultures due to their potential therapeutic benefits. Botanicals like uva-ursi, marshmallow root, and corn silk are thought to have anti-inflammatory and antimicrobial properties that may help to relieve the symptoms of cystitis. These remedies are believed to synergistically work with the body to promote overall health while addressing the particular problems associated with cystitis.

Alternative therapies are another facet of holistic approaches to treating cystitis. Acupuncture, for example, has drawn attention for its ability to adjust the body's energy flow and boost the immune system, which may help resolve the condition. Similarly, chiropractic adjustments and osteopathic manipulative treatments target the restoration of musculoskeletal balance in an effort to improve the body's self-healing capabilities. These alternative therapies emphasize a holistic perspective of the patient, taking into account not only the symptoms but also the person's general health and way of life.

Mind-body techniques are an essential part of holistic approaches to treating cystitis.

The interconnection of mental and physical well-being emphasizes the importance of addressing psychological aspects in the management of cystitis. Deep breathing exercises, mindfulness meditation, and biofeedback are some of the techniques that aim to mitigate the effects of chronic stress and emotional factors on cystitis symptoms. Also, by promoting relaxation and stress reduction, these techniques may help improve the patient's overall quality of life and alleviate symptoms.

Together, herbal remedies, alternative therapies, and mind-body techniques make up a comprehensive approach to treating cystitis that takes into account the patient's physical, mental, and emotional well-being. Including these holistic modalities in the management of cystitis represents a paradigm shift towards personalized and patient-centered care, recognizing the complexity of factors influencing health and healing.

Natural Treatments For Cystitis

For centuries, people have used herbal remedies to treat a variety of illnesses, including cystitis. One such herb that has been used traditionally for its potential antimicrobial properties is uva-ursi, also known as bearberry. The active compound, arbutin, is thought to convert into hydroquinone, exhibiting antibacterial effects and possibly reducing bacterial colonization in the bladder. Another herbal remedy that is well-known for its soothing and anti-inflammatory properties is marshmallow root; by reducing inflammation in the bladder lining, it may help relieve the discomfort that comes with cystitis. Finally, corn silk, which is made from the silky fibers found on corn cobs, is believed to have diuretic properties

Herbal remedies have the potential to be beneficial, but it is important to use caution when using them. The effectiveness of these remedies can vary, and it is important to take into account any interactions with medications. Additionally, speaking with a healthcare provider is necessary to confirm that herbal treatments are suitable for specific cases of cystitis. Herbal remedies can be used in conjunction with conventional medical treatments as a complementary measure, giving patients more options for managing their condition and enhancing their overall health.

Alternative Cystitis Treatments

Acupuncture, a traditional Chinese medicine practice, involves the insertion of thin needles into specific points on the body to stimulate energy flow. In the context of cystitis, acupuncture is thought to balance the body's energy, potentially enhancing the immune response and promoting overall bladder health. Chiropractic care and osteopathic manipulative treatments focus on the musculoskeletal system, aiming to restore alignment and improve the body's ability to self-heal. These alternative therapies have a significant role in the holistic management of cystitis because they offer diverse approaches beyond conventional medical interventions. They also highlight the interconnectedness of various bodily systems and provide a customized approach to cystitis management.

While alternative therapies are promising, it is important to recognize that individual differences in efficacy may exist, and the scientific evidence for their use in treating cystitis is still being developed. Moreover, incorporating alternative therapies into the care of patients with cystitis should be done in consultation with a healthcare provider who can evaluate each patient's suitability for them. Finally, the holistic nature of alternative therapies is consistent with the comprehensive approach to managing cystitis, which emphasizes the importance of treating not only symptoms but also the patient's overall health and lifestyle.

Mind-Body Methods For Treating Cystitis

The integration of mind-body techniques into the comprehensive management of cystitis is important because it acknowledges the complex relationship between mental and physical health. As emotional and chronic stress can exacerbate the symptoms of cystitis, mind-body techniques are an essential part of comprehensive care. Mindfulness meditation, which focuses on the present moment and mindfulness, has been shown to be effective in lowering stress and improving mental health in general.

Deep breathing exercises, like diaphragmatic breathing, can cause a relaxation response, which can help release tension and stress that may aggravate cystitis symptoms.

The application of biofeedback, a therapeutic modality that permits individuals to monitor and regulate physiological processes, has been investigated in relation to the management of cystitis. Through the provision of real-time physiological function information, biofeedback enables individuals to take charge of specific bodily reactions, which may have an impact on the intensity of symptoms associated with cystitis. These mind-body approaches highlight the significance of incorporating psychological elements into the comprehensive treatment plan for cystitis, recognizing the reciprocal relationship between mental and physical health.

In summary, the integration of mind-body techniques into the holistic management of cystitis recognizes the interdependence of mental and physical health. Through the identification and treatment of stress and emotional factors, these techniques serve to enhance overall health and quality of life for cystitis patients beyond symptom management.

CHAPTER FIVE
UNDERSTANDING CURRENT CYSTITIES

Because recurrent cystitis is a common urinary tract infection (UTI) that primarily affects women, it requires a thorough understanding in order to effectively manage and prevent its recurrence. Cystitis, which is characterized by inflammation of the bladder, can be caused by a variety of bacteria, with Escherichia coli being the predominant pathogen. In order to develop targeted interventions, it is important to understand the anatomical and physiological factors that contribute to recurrent cystitis. Women are more vulnerable to bacterial invasion because of their shorter urethra than men, and because of this, women are more likely to experience recurrent episodes due to this condition. Additionally, hormonal fluctuations, particularly during menopause, can alter the urogenital microbiota, creating an environment that is favorable to bacterial coloni

Recognizing Triggers

Finding triggers is essential to treating recurrent cystitis. Triggers can be behavioral, environmental, or physiological. Behavioral triggers include things like wiping from back to front, which can introduce bacteria into the urethra; sexual activity is another major behavioral trigger, and it's important to understand how it affects the recurrence of cystitis. Lifestyle factors, like diet, stress, and smoking, can also increase the risk of recurrent infections. Environmental triggers include things like exposure to irritants or allergens, underscoring the significance of treating patients holistically. Physiological factors include anatomical abnormalities or underlying medical conditions

Preventive Actions

Preventive measures play a pivotal role in managing and mitigating the recurrence of cystitis. Education on proper hygiene practices, including wiping techniques and adequate genital care, is fundamental. Behavioral modifications, such as avoiding irritants like harsh soaps or feminine hygiene products, contribute to a reduced risk of recurrent infections. Hydration is a key preventive measure, as it promotes frequent urination, flushing out bacteria from the urinary tract. Lifestyle changes, including a balanced diet and stress management, can strengthen the immune system, making the body more resilient to infections. Prophylactic antibiotic therapy may be considered in certain cases, although this approach requires careful consideration of potential risks and benefits. Exploring alternative and complementary therapies, such as probiotics or herbal supplements, adds a dimension to preventive strategies.

A comprehensive, multidisciplinary approach ensures a well-rounded and personalized preventive plan tailored to the individual's unique risk factors.

Looking for Expert Medical Attention:

In cases of recurrent cystitis, seeking specialized care becomes imperative to address the underlying causes and ensure effective management. Consulting a urologist or a specialist in female urology is essential for a thorough evaluation, including imaging studies and urodynamic tests. Urodynamic assessments help identify any structural or functional abnormalities that may contribute to recurrent infections. Additionally, specialized care involves a detailed medical history review, considering previous episodes, treatments, and the patient's overall health. For postmenopausal women, hormonal therapy may be explored to restore the urogenital microbiota and reduce the risk of recurrence. In cases where anatomic abnormalities are identified, surgical interventions may be recommended to correct predisposing factors.

Furthermore, a collaborative approach with gynecologists and infectious disease specialists ensures a comprehensive evaluation and tailored management plan. Patient education regarding the importance of follow-up and adherence to treatment plans is integral to the success of specialized care in recurrent cystitis.

CHAPTER SIX
CYSTITIES IN PARTICULAR POPULATIONS

Cystitis in women is a prevalent and often recurrent urinary tract infection (UTI) characterized by inflammation of the bladder lining, usually caused by bacterial infection, with Escherichia coli (E. coli) being a common culprit. Women are more susceptible to cystitis due to their shorter urethra, which facilitates easier entry of bacteria into the bladder. The anatomical proximity of the urethra to the anus further increases the risk of bacterial migration. Hormonal factors, such as changes in estrogen levels, pregnancy, and the use of certain contraceptives, may also contribute to the vulnerability of women to cystitis. Symptoms often include dysuria, frequent urination, and a sense of urgency. Diagnosis is typically based on clinical presentation, urinalysis, and, if necessary, urine culture.

Treatment involves antibiotic therapy, hydration, and measures to alleviate symptoms.

Prevention strategies, including proper hygiene, urination habits, and cranberry products, are crucial in managing and preventing recurrent cystitis in women.

Men's Cystitis

While cystitis is more commonly associated with women, it can also affect men, although less frequently. Men are generally at a lower risk due to the longer length of their urethra, which acts as a barrier to bacterial entry. When cystitis occurs in men, it often raises concerns about underlying urinary tract abnormalities or compromised immune function. In men, cystitis is more commonly associated with conditions such as an enlarged prostate or urethral stricture. Additionally, men who engage in anal intercourse may be at an increased risk of bacterial migration. The symptoms of cystitis in men are similar to those in women and may include dysuria, frequency, and urgency.

Diagnosis involves a thorough medical history, physical examination, and relevant laboratory tests. Treatment typically includes a course of antibiotics tailored to the specific pathogen. Addressing underlying factors contributing to cystitis in men is essential for preventing recurrence. While cystitis is less common in men, understanding its etiology and prompt intervention are crucial for effective management.

Cystitis In Children

Pediatric cystitis refers to bladder inflammation in children, which can present unique challenges in terms of diagnosis and management. In children, cystitis may manifest with nonspecific symptoms such as abdominal pain, changes in behavior, and fever, making it essential for healthcare providers to maintain a high index of suspicion. The causes of cystitis in children are diverse and can include bacterial infections, structural abnormalities, or voiding dysfunction.

Girls are more commonly affected than boys in the pediatric population, mirroring the gender prevalence observed in adults. Diagnosis often involves a combination of clinical evaluation, urinalysis, and urine culture. Treatment includes antibiotics, and in some cases, imaging studies may be required to assess for any anatomical abnormalities. Pediatric cystitis management requires a tailored approach, considering the child's age, potential underlying causes, and the choice of appropriate antibiotics. Educating parents about preventive measures, such as proper hygiene and encouraging fluid intake, is vital for reducing the risk of recurrence in pediatric cystitis.

CHAPTER SEVEN
HANDLING CHRONIC CYSTITIS

The challenge of managing chronic cystitis encompasses not only the physical symptoms but also the substantial emotional and psychological effects it can have on individuals. The recurrent nature of the condition frequently results in frustration, anxiety, and a reduced quality of life for patients. The ongoing discomfort and unpredictable flare-ups can also contribute to a feeling of helplessness. Social stigma surrounding urinary issues can also exacerbate feelings of embarrassment and isolation. Patients may find it difficult to talk about their condition honestly, which exacerbates the emotional load. Consequently, coping strategies for chronic cystitis must address both the physical and emotional aspects of the condition.

Peer support groups and online communities can also offer a valuable space for people to share experiences, reducing the sense of isolation often associated with chronic health conditions. Psychosocial interventions, such as cognitive-behavioral therapy, can help individuals develop effective coping mechanisms and resilience in the face of chronic cystitis. Healthcare professionals play a crucial role in supporting patients through education and counseling. Providing a thorough understanding of the condition, its triggers, and management options can empower patients to take an active role in their care.

Adopting lifestyle changes is another important part of managing chronic cystitis. Stress reduction methods, like mindfulness and relaxation exercises, can be helpful because stress is known to aggravate cystitis symptoms. Keeping hydrated, eating a healthy diet, and engaging in regular exercise can also improve general wellbeing and possibly reduce symptoms. By addressing the psychological, emotional, and lifestyle aspects of chronic cystitis, people can improve their capacity to manage the difficulties it presents.

Impact On Emotion And Psychology

The recurrent and often unpredictable nature of chronic cystitis can have a significant emotional and psychological impact on those who are affected. The condition can significantly disrupt daily activities and interpersonal relationships, which can lead to feelings of frustration, helplessness, and even depression.

Patients may experience elevated levels of stress and anxiety due to the constant physical discomfort and the possibility of acute flare-ups. Additionally, social withdrawal and a lower quality of life may result from the fear of embarrassment associated with urinary symptoms.

A holistic approach, acknowledging the emotional aspects of the condition alongside its physical manifestations, is necessary for healthcare providers to develop comprehensive care strategies. Psychosocial support, such as counseling and mental health interventions, should be integrated into the overall management plan. Patients benefit from having a safe space to express their concerns, fears, and frustrations, fostering a sense of validation and understanding.

A more comprehensive and patient-centered approach to care can be achieved by addressing the emotional and psychological aspects of chronic cystitis. Self-help strategies, in addition to professional support, are essential for managing the emotional and psychological impact of the condition. Mindfulness-based techniques, like meditation and deep breathing exercises, can help people cope with stress and anxiety.

Education about the condition and its triggers can empower patients to proactively manage their symptoms and reduce the emotional burden.

Assistive Techniques

Supportive strategies are essential for improving the general quality of life for people with chronic cystitis. They are multimodal in nature, addressing the emotional as well as the physical symptoms of the condition. Support can be obtained from a variety of sources, such as social networks, medical professionals, and self-help interventions.

Effective supportive care is built on the foundation of a strong doctor-patient relationship. Healthcare providers play a central role in providing support through clear communication, education, and personalized treatment plans. Giving patients knowledge about cystitis, its triggers, and available management options empowers them to actively participate in their care. Regular follow-up appointments offer an opportunity for ongoing support and modifications to treatment plans based on individual responses and needs.

Social support is just as important for people with chronic cystitis.

Getting involved with friends, family, or support groups can help reduce the feelings of loneliness that come with having a chronic illness.

Peer support enables people to talk about their experiences, coping mechanisms, and emotional struggles, which creates a sense of community. Online forums and communities specifically for people with cystitis offer a useful forum for people to interact and share knowledge.

Self-help strategies are an adjunct to professional and social support. Individuals with chronic cystitis can create a comprehensive support system that improves their overall well-being by combining professional guidance, social support, and personalized self-help strategies. Developing personalized coping mechanisms, such as keeping a symptom diary, practicing stress management techniques, and adopting a healthy lifestyle, empowers people to actively manage their condition.

Including Cystitis Management In Everyday Activities

In order to effectively manage chronic cystitis, people must incorporate strategies that work into their daily lives in order to help them feel in control and normal despite the obstacles that the condition presents. These strategies can take many different forms, such as treatment adherence, lifestyle modifications, and proactive symptom management.

The attainment of optimal outcomes in the management of cystitis is contingent upon adherence to treatment plans. Healthcare providers are pivotal in guaranteeing that individuals comprehend the prescription medications, possible side effects, and the significance of consistent use. The incorporation of medication into daily routines, such as associating its administration with regular activities, can bolster adherence. Frequent follow-up appointments afford healthcare providers the chance to evaluate the efficacy of treatment and make any necessary modifications, thereby fostering continuous engagement in the management process.

A routine that includes drinking enough water, eating a balanced diet, and exercising regularly supports overall wellbeing. Stress management techniques, when skillfully integrated into daily activities, can lessen the impact of stress on cystitis symptoms. Identifying and avoiding triggers, such as certain foods or activities, contributes to symptom control.

Increasing body awareness and spotting early warning signs of flare-ups are important components of proactive symptom management. Keeping a symptom diary can help people keep track of triggers and patterns, which will help them anticipate and manage possible exacerbations. Being proactive allows people to take immediate action, such as rest, increased fluid intake, or other customized strategies, to reduce the impact of cystitis symptoms on day-to-day activities.

As a result, despite the difficulties presented by chronic cystitis, people can regain a sense of control and normalcy by addressing treatment adherence, lifestyle modifications, and proactive symptom management. Healthcare providers, support networks, and self-help strategies all work together to create a holistic framework that enables people to successfully navigate the challenges of living with this condition. In conclusion, the successful integration of cystitis management into daily life requires a comprehensive and personalized approach.

Research And Treatment Advancements For Cystitis

Cystitis, an inflammation of the bladder usually brought on by a bacterial infection, has long been a medical problem. Many studies have been carried out to determine the pathophysiology of cystitis and to devise strategies for treatment. One major area of research has been the investigation of novel diagnostic techniques in an effort to improve early detection and accurate identification of the causative agents. The use of modern molecular techniques, such as PCR and advanced imaging modalities, has made diagnosis more precise and has made timely interventions possible.

Within the field of pharmacotherapy, the creation of new antimicrobial agents and antibiotic classes has been of utmost importance. Scientists have been investigating new drug classes and combinations to address the issue of antibiotic resistance, which is becoming more and more prevalent in the treatment of cystitis. Moreover, efforts have been focused on optimizing current antibiotics, enhancing their effectiveness and mitigating side effects.

The application of nanotechnology in drug delivery systems presents opportunities for targeted and sustained release, which could potentially transform the way antimicrobial agents are administered.

As researchers explore the complex interactions between the immune system and cystitis, they have become more interested in immunotherapeutic approaches. Vaccination strategies, which make use of knowledge about bacterial virulence factors, are designed to elicit a strong immune response and offer long-term protection against recurring infections. Another area of research involves developing immunomodulatory drugs to improve the innate immune response. These developments highlight the dynamic character of cystitis research, as there is constant effort to improve treatment modalities and meet the condition's ever-changing challenges.

Current Studies In Medicine

The current body of medical research on cystitis has surpassed the limitations of traditional treatment approaches by integrating a thorough understanding of the host-pathogen interactions and the bladder microenvironment. Researchers are examining the impact of the urinary tract microbiome on immune modulation and the development of chronic cystitis, with the goal of identifying microbial signatures associated with disease progression. The microbiome of the urinary tract has emerged as a critical factor influencing susceptibility to cystitis and response to treatment.

In addition, novel biomarkers for early diagnosis and prognosis assessment have been identified thanks to the integration of big data analytics and artificial intelligence. These state-of-the-art technologies offer a paradigm shift in the understanding and management of cystitis and usher in an era of precision medicine. Genetic factors influencing susceptibility to infections and drug metabolism are under scrutiny, guiding the development of tailored therapeutic strategies.

In addition to traditional pharmacological interventions, non-pharmacological modalities such as physical therapy, dietary changes, and lifestyle interventions are being studied for their ability to reduce symptoms and avoid recurrent infections.

Integrative approaches, which take into account the whole health of people with cystitis, are becoming more and more popular, highlighting the significance of interdisciplinary cooperation in the field of medical research.

New Therapies

Regarding novel treatments for cystitis, research on adjunctive and alternative therapies has gained traction. Probiotics, which have the ability to repair and preserve a healthy urinary microbiome, are being studied as a preventative and therapeutic measure.

Studies on the effectiveness of particular probiotic strains in preventing recurrent infections and regulating immune responses in the urinary tract are currently in progress.

Aiming to reduce the risk of catheter-associated infections, nanomaterials with inherent antimicrobial properties are being explored as coatings for urinary catheters.

Nanoparticles loaded with antimicrobial agents can enhance drug penetration into the bladder tissues, improving therapeutic outcomes while minimizing side effects.

Nanotechnology, with its ability to manipulate materials at the molecular and nanoscale levels, is opening new frontiers in drug delivery for cystitis treatment.

In addition to antimicrobials, researchers are examining the role of anti-inflammatory agents in the management of cystitis. By focusing on the inflammatory pathways that underlie the symptoms and complications of cystitis, these therapies seek to both relieve symptoms and stop the condition from getting worse. Immunomodulatory drugs, on the other hand, are being studied for their potential to modulate the host's defense mechanisms against bacterial invasion.

Prospective Courses

Researchers, clinicians, and industry stakeholders must work together to translate scientific discoveries into clinically meaningful advancements in cystitis treatment and research. Future directions of cystitis research and treatment will take a multifaceted approach that addresses not only the microbial factors but also the host's immune response, genetic predispositions, and environmental influences.

The combination of systems biology and multi-omics approaches holds promise for deciphering the complexities of cystitis and paving the way for more targeted and effective interventions.

Technological developments in telemedicine and digital health are expected to have a significant impact on how cystitis is managed in the future. Technologies such as teleconsultations, mobile health applications, and remote monitoring may improve patient participation, enable prompt interventions, and supply important data for continued research. Artificial intelligence algorithms that can process large amounts of data could be useful in forecasting the course of the disease, making treatment recommendations, and locating new therapeutic targets.

It is anticipated that patient-centered care and shared decision-making will become more prevalent, recognizing the various experiences and preferences of people with cystitis. Future approaches will likely include customizing treatment plans to patients' specific needs while taking psychosocial factors and quality of life into account. Providing patients with self-management techniques and education may improve outcomes and lessen the burden of recurring infections.

CONCLUSION

the path to curing cystitis is characterized by a dynamic interaction between research, developments, and future paths. The changing face of cystitis treatment demonstrates a dedication to creativity and a comprehensive comprehension of the ailment.

From delving into the complexities of the urinary microbiome to utilizing nanotechnology and immunotherapy, the field keeps pushing the envelope.

New therapeutics like probiotics and nanomedicine offer fresh ways to tackle the problems of antibiotic resistance and recurrent infections. Looking ahead, multifaceted approaches that combine systems biology, digital health technologies, and patient-centered care are set to transform cystitis management. Current medical research has established the groundwork for personalized medicine in cystitis treatment, with genomics, big data analytics, and artificial intelligence defining a new era of precision healthcare.

Together, clinicians, researchers, industry partners, and most importantly, the people impacted by the condition must work together to conquer cystitis.

Through a relentless pursuit of knowledge, technological innovation, and a dedication to patient care, the medical community is in a position to revolutionize the management of cystitis and enhance the lives of those who suffer from this common but difficult urinary tract condition.

www.ingramcontent.com/pod-product-compliance
Lightning Source LLC
Chambersburg PA
CBHW071129260726